STOMACH ULCER

PROFESSIONAL APPROACH TO STOMACH
ULCER

DR. J. WALLER

Contents

INTRODUCTION 3

CHAPTER ONE 5

Definition of Stomach Ulcers 5

Frequency and Effect on Intestinal Health.............................7

Comprehending Ulcers of the Stomach 12

Signs and a diagnosis 18

CHAPTER TWO 19

Methods of treating stomach ulcers..................................25

Problems and Prolonged Handling....................................31

Nutritional Aspects 38

CHAPTER THREE 43

Modifications to Lifestyle..46

Emotional Health and Coping Mechanisms 52

CHAPTER FOUR 58

Avoidance...59

CONCLUSION...65

THE END 68

INTRODUCTION

Open sores that form on the stomach lining are called gastric ulcers or stomach ulcers. These ulcers are also known as duodenal ulcers when they develop in the duodenum, the top portion of the small intestine. Peptic ulcers, of which stomach ulcers are a kind, can result in pain, discomfort, and other symptoms.

The imbalance between the stomach's defenses and the things that can harm its lining is frequently associated with the development of stomach ulcers. The presence of the bacteria Helicobacter pylori (H. pylori), long-term use of nonsteroidal anti-inflammatory medicines (NSAIDs), excessive production of stomach acid, and lifestyle variables like stress and smoking can all have an impact on this imbalance.

Stomach ulcer symptoms might include burning pain in the stomach, bloating, nausea, vomiting, and in more serious cases, complications such as bleeding or stomach lining perforation.

accurate diagnosis and treatment, which frequently includes taking antibiotics for H. pylori and drugs to lower stomach acid. Eliminating the pylori bacteria and making lifestyle changes are crucial for controlling and curing stomach ulcers. In order to avoid problems and encourage recovery, early detection and action are essential.

CHAPTER ONE

Definition of Stomach Ulcers

Peptic ulcers, also referred to as stomach ulcers, are open sores that develop on the duodenum, the top portion of the small intestine, or the inside lining of the stomach. These ulcers develop when the duodenum's or stomach's protective lining erodes, exposing underlying tissues to stomach acids.

The main causes of stomach ulcers include excess stomach acid production, long-term use of nonsteroidal anti-inflammatory medicines (NSAIDs), such as aspirin or ibuprofen, and Helicobacter pylori (H. pylori) infection. Certain medical disorders, heavy alcohol intake, and smoking could all be additional contributing factors.

A burning or painful feeling in the stomach, bloating, nausea, and vomiting are just a few of the symptoms that can be caused by stomach ulcers. Severe problems could include bleeding, duodenal or stomach perforations, or blockage.

Antibiotics are often used to eradicate H and medicines are used to lower stomach acid in the management and treatment of stomach ulcers. alterations in lifestyle, if there is a pylori infection. In order to avoid problems and encourage the healing of the ulcerated areas, prompt action is essential.

Frequency and Effect on Intestinal Health

In recent decades, there has been a decline in the prevalence of stomach ulcers, partly due to improved understanding of their origins and the development of efficient therapies. Still, they have a major global impact on a large number of people.

Occurrence:

H. pylori Infection:

One important cause of stomach ulcers is the bacterium Helicobacter pylori, sometimes known as H. pylori. More than half of people on the planet are thought to be H-infected. pylori. But not every person with H. pylori causes ulcers, however there are additional contributing factors.

Gender and Age:

Although they can happen to anyone at any age, stomach ulcers are more prevalent in older persons. Compared to women, men are more likely to get stomach ulcers.

Usage of NSAIDs:

Aspirin and ibuprofen are two examples of nonsteroidal anti-inflammatory drug (NSAID) long-term use that significantly increases the risk of stomach ulcers. NSAID use is common for a variety of medical ailments, which raises the risk of ulcers.

Effect on the Digestive System:

Gastric Lining Disruption:

The protective lining of the duodenum or stomach is disrupted as a result of stomach ulcers. Pain, suffering, and problems may result from this.

Manifestations and Life Quality:

The presence of stomach ulcer symptoms, such as bloating, nausea, and abdominal discomfort, can seriously impair a person's quality of life. Chronic illnesses might influence daily activities and food choices.

Problems:

Serious consequences from stomach ulcers include bleeding, duodenal or stomach perforation, and obstruction of the gastric outlet if treatment is not received. These issues need to be treated right away because they may be fatal.

Effect on Uptake of Nutrients:

Nutrient shortages may arise from stomach ulcers obstructing the body's ability to absorb nutrients. This may worsen existing health problems and have an impact on general wellbeing.

Effect on the Mind:

Stress and worry might be psychological effects of having stomach ulcers. In turn, stress has the potential to worsen symptoms and impede the healing process.

Outlook and Management:

With the proper medical assistance, such as drugs to lower stomach acid and antibiotics for H. Most stomach ulcers can be effectively cured with pylori removal and lifestyle changes.

In order to avoid problems and encourage the healing of ulcerated regions, early detection and treatment are essential.

Adopting a balanced diet, reducing stress, and staying away from NSAIDs are just a few examples of lifestyle modifications that can help stop stomach ulcers from recurring.

Those who exhibit symptoms that could indicate stomach ulcers should get medical help as soon as possible to ensure a proper diagnosis and course of treatment. It's critical to follow up with medical professionals on a regular basis to assess progress and modify treatment programs as necessary.

Comprehending Ulcers of the Stomach

Investigating the causes, signs, diagnosis, and treatment of stomach ulcers is necessary to comprehend them. Now let's examine the main features of stomach ulcers:

Reasons:

H. pylori Infection:

One of the most prevalent causes of stomach ulcers is the bacteria Helicobacter pylori, or H. pylori. It makes the stomach's lining less strong and more vulnerable to the damaging effects of stomach acids.

Usage of NSAIDs:

Nonsteroidal anti-inflammatory medicines (NSAIDs), such ibuprofen and aspirin, can irritate the stomach lining over time and increase the risk of ulcer development.

Too Much Stomach Acid

Ulcers can result from the overproduction of stomach acid, which erodes the mucous lining.

Alcohol and Smoking:

There is a link between smoking and binge drinking and a higher risk of stomach ulcers.

Stress

Although stress does not directly cause ulcers, it can aggravate their symptoms and slow down their healing.

Signs:

Burning Anguish:

an abdominal ache or burning feeling, especially at night and in between meals.

Belching and Bloating:

feeling bloated and frequently spitting up.

vomiting and nauseous:

vomiting and nausea, with or without blood in it.

Unexpected Loss of Weight:

Significant loss of weight for which there is no obvious cause.

Black Barstools:

dark, tarry stools are present, which could be a sign of ulcer bleeding.

Upper Endoscopy:

A frequent technique that involves seeing within the stomach and duodenum with an endoscope— a thin, flexible tube equipped with a camera.

Barium X-ray:

A series of X-rays that are obtained after the patient consumes a barium solution, enabling the stomach and duodenum to be seen.

Tests for Stool and Blood:

blood examinations to identify H. stool tests and pylori antibodies to detect the presence of blood.

Therapy:

Drugs:

H2 blockers and proton pump inhibitors (PPIs) help lessen the production of stomach acid.

drugs to get rid of H. pylori infection.

Anthems:

Antacids available over-the-counter to relieve symptoms.

Modifications in Lifestyle:

avoiding NSAIDs, giving up smoking, consuming less alcohol, and controlling stress.

Dietary Adjustments:

consuming a diet that lessens the creation of stomach acid and encourages recovery.

Problems:

Bleeding Ulcers:

Bleeding from ulcers can result in anemia and black stools.

Breach:

Ulcers are rare but dangerous because they can pierce the duodenum or stomach wall.

Blockage of the Gastric Outlet:

Long-term ulceration scarring might make it difficult for food to exit the stomach.

Comprehending gastric ulcers entails identifying potential risk factors, being cognizant of symptoms, obtaining prompt medical assistance, and actively engaging in an all-encompassing treatment regimen. Most people with stomach ulcers are able to recover and avoid problems with the right care. It's critical to follow up with medical professionals on a regular basis to assess progress and modify treatment plans as necessary.

Signs and a diagnosis

Peptic ulcers, another name for stomach ulcers, can present with a variety of symptoms, and diagnosing them requires a number of different medical evaluations.

CHAPTER TWO

The following list of typical signs and procedures for diagnosing stomach ulcers:

Signs:

Burning Anguish:

an abdominal ache or burning feeling that usually occurs at night and in between meals.

Belching and Bloating:

feeling bloated and frequently spitting up.

vomiting and nauseous:

intermittent vomiting, sometimes with blood in it, and nausea.

Unexpected Loss of Weight:

Notable loss of weight without a clear reason.

Black Barstools:

dark, tarry stools are present, which could be a sign of ulcer bleeding.

Heartburn:

persistent heartburn, especially if antacids purchased over-the-counter do not reduce the pain.

discomfort following a meal:

soreness or discomfort in the upper abdomen following a meal.

Upper Endoscopy:

a typical treatment that involves seeing within the stomach and duodenum with an endoscopea thin, flexible tube equipped with a camera. Tissue samples (biopsies) can be obtained during an endoscopy for additional analysis.

Barium X-ray:

After the patient consumes a barium solution, X-rays are obtained to visualize the duodenum and stomach. This test can identify locations that have ulcers.

Blood Examinations:

It is possible to perform blood tests to determine whether H is present. pylori antibodies or indications of hemorrhagic ulcer anemia.

Stool Examinations:

Blood can be seen in stool tests, which may indicate bleeding from the duodenum or stomach.

H. pylori examinations:

tests to look for the bacteria Helicobacter pylori, also known as H. pylori, which is connected to stomach ulcers. A blood test, breath test, or biopsy during an endoscopy may be required for this.

MRI or CT scan:

Imaging techniques, including an MRI or CT scan, can be utilized to determine complications and determine the amount of ulceration.

Analyzing the stomach:

A gastric analysis may be done in certain situations to gauge the stomach's acid production.

Endoscopic Sonography (EUS):

This produces finely detailed images of the stomach wall and surrounding structures by combining endoscopy and ultrasonography.

Observation and Investigation:

Recheck Endoscopy:

When it comes to H. pylori infection, a follow-up endoscopy might be suggested to verify the bacteria's elimination and track the healing of the ulcer.

Continual Imaging:

Imaging scans can be carried out on a regular basis to track ulcer healing and identify any problems.

Keeping an eye on symptoms:

Symptoms should be regularly monitored to evaluate the efficacy of treatment.

Effective treatments for stomach ulcers include medication, dietary modifications, and, in H. antibiotics and pylori infection. It's essential to follow up with medical professionals on a regular basis to assess treatment outcomes, track advancements, and handle any potential issues.

Medication, lifestyle changes, and, in certain situations, treating the underlying reasons are all part of the treatment for stomach ulcers. The following are typical methods for treating stomach ulcers:

Drugs:

PPIs, or proton pump inhibitors:

Drugs that lower stomach acid production, such as omeprazole, esomeprazole, and lansoprazole, promote ulcer healing. Usually, a prescription for these lasts a few weeks.

H2 Blockers:

Ranitidine and famotidine are examples of histamine-2 (H2) blockers that lower stomach acid and encourage the healing of ulcers.

Anthems:

Antacids sold over-the-counter neutralize stomach acid to produce immediate relief. They can aid in symptom management but do not support long-term recovery.

Agents Cytoprotective:

Sucralfate and other similar medications coat the ulcer to promote healing and stop additional damage.

Antibiotics:

A cocktail of antibiotics, including amoxicillin, clarithromycin, and metronidazole, is administered to remove Helicobacter pylori (H. pylori) if it is the cause of the ulcer.

Changes in Lifestyle:

Modifications to Diet:

Reducing irritation to the stomach lining can be achieved by avoiding foods that are spicy, acidic, or irritating. It might also be advantageous to eat smaller, more frequent meals.

Give Up Smoking:

Smoking raises the possibility of complications and can slow the healing of ulcers. It's advised to give up smoking.

Limit Consumption of Alcohol:

The stomach lining may get irritated by excessive alcohol drinking. Reducing alcohol consumption could help ulcers heal.

Handling Stress:

Although stress doesn't directly cause ulcers, it can make them worse. Counseling and other stress-reduction methods like relaxation training could be helpful.

Steer clear of NSAIDs:

Avoid or use nonsteroidal anti-inflammatory medicines (NSAIDs) sparingly if at all feasible, as they may exacerbate the development of ulcers.

Recheck Endoscopy:

Tracking the Healing Process:

To track the ulcer's healing, a follow-up endoscopy can be advised, particularly if the initial diagnosis included problems.

H. pylori examination:

Should H. If a pylori infection was the reason, more testing might be carried out to make sure the bacterium was successfully eradicated.

Surgery: Infrequent Cases

Problems:

Surgical intervention may be required in cases of significant bleeding, perforation, or obstruction of the stomach outlet.

Durable Ulcers:

Surgical options like antrectomy or vagotomy may be explored if ulcers don't go away or keep coming back.

Continuous Administration:

Frequent Check-ins:

It's critical to schedule routine check-ups with medical professionals to evaluate ulcer healing progress, modify medication, and handle any new concerns.

Extended-term Drugs:

Long-term usage of drugs like PPIs may be advised in some circumstances, particularly for people with a history of recurrent ulcers or persistent risk factors.

Those who have stomach ulcers should make sure they adhere to their doctor's recommended course of action, keep all of their follow-up appointments, and let them know if their symptoms change or cause them concern. A successful recovery and the avoidance of problems are facilitated by good management and strict adherence to the treatment plan.

Problems and Prolonged Handling

Complications may arise from poorly managed or untreated stomach ulcers. The goal of long-term care is to address the underlying causes of ulcer formation and avoid recurrence. The following are possible side effects and long-term care techniques:

Problems:

Bleeding Ulcers:

Internal bleeding from ulcers can result in anemia and, in extreme situations, necessitate immediate medical intervention.

Breach:

Rarely, ulcers can pierce the duodenum or stomach, resulting in peritonitis, a potentially fatal illness that needs to be treated right away with surgery.

Blockage of the Gastric Outlet:

Long-term ulceration scarring can hinder food exiting the stomach, leading to nausea, vomiting, and weight loss.

Extended-Term Administration:

Adherence to Medication:

Following the prescription for drugs like H2 blockers or proton pump inhibitors (PPIs) is essential for minimizing acid-related damage and accelerating ulcer healing.

H. pylori Elimination:

Should H. Since the presence of pylori infection was a contributing factor, it is imperative to finish the recommended course of antibiotics and undergo further testing to ensure eradication.

Steer Clear of Triggering Substances:

Long-term ulcer therapy requires ongoing avoidance of medications that can irritate the stomach lining, such as NSAIDs.

Changes in Lifestyle:

Maintaining a healthy lifestyle that includes regular exercise, a balanced diet, and stress reduction will help avoid ulcer recurrence and enhance general wellbeing.

Frequent Endoscopy Follow-up:

It could be advised to do periodic endoscopies to track the ulcer's healing and look for any indications of problems or recurrence.

Handling of Difficulties:

Timely medical attention and action are critical in the event of complications such as bleeding or perforation. Hospitalization and, in extreme situations, surgery may be necessary for this.

Quitting Smoking:

Since smoking can impede the healing process, giving up is good for general health and ulcer healing.

Reducing Alcohol Consumption:

Limiting alcohol intake aids in lessening stomach lining inflammation.

Handling Tension:

Long-term ulcer management may benefit from using stress-reduction strategies like counseling or relaxation exercises.

Support for Nutrition:

Nutritional support could be required in situations when there is weight loss or nutritional deficits. A well-balanced diet that promotes healing can be created with the assistance of a dietician.

Knowledge and Consciousness:

It is important to inform patients about the warning signals of an ulcer recurrence and to get medical help if symptoms intensify or resurface.

Continuous Observation:

Frequent Examinations:

For the purpose of resolving any new concerns, modifying medication, and assessing the efficacy of the treatment plan, routine check-ups with medical professionals are crucial.

Patient Instruction:

Encouraging patients to make lifestyle changes and long-term management a priority is crucial to enabling them to take an active role in their health care.

A cooperative effort between patients and healthcare professionals is necessary for effective long-term therapy in order to control problems, avoid recurrence, and enhance general gastrointestinal health. Successful, long-term ulcer management is facilitated by regular follow-ups and communication.

Nutritional Aspects

By encouraging healing, lowering discomfort, and minimizing recurrence of symptoms, dietary considerations are essential in the management of stomach ulcers. Although dietary responses to particular foods may differ across individuals, the following are basic guidelines for those who have stomach ulcers:

Foods to Add:

High-Fibre Foods:

Legumes, fruits, vegetables, and whole grains all offer vital nutrients and support a healthy digestive system.

Trim Proteins:

Lean protein sources that are less likely to upset the stomach include beans, fish, fowl, and tofu.

Low-Satin Milk:

Select dairy products that are low in fat or fat free to avoid too much fat, which can increase the formation of stomach acid.

Produce and Fruits:

The majority of fruits and vegetables include vital vitamins and antioxidants and are generally well-tolerated. If acidic varieties cause symptoms, steer clear of them.

Good Fats:

Incorporate moderate amounts of foods high in healthful fats, such as almonds, avocados, and olive oil.

Probiotics:

Foods high in probiotics, such as yogurt made with living cultures, can improve intestinal health.

Fish in Cold Water:

Omega-3 fatty acids are abundant in cold-water fish, such as mackerel and salmon, and they may have anti-inflammatory properties.

Herbal Teas:

Herbal teas without caffeine, such chamomile or ginger tea, can be calming.

Foods to Steer Clear of:

Hot Foods:

Spicy foods and spices might aggravate symptoms by irritating the stomach lining.

Fruits with Citrus Flavors:

Acidic fruits such as tomatoes, oranges, and grapefruits should be consumed in moderation as they may cause discomfort.

Products Made From Tomatoes:

Products and sauces made from tomatoes can be unpleasant and acidic.

Coffee:

Coffee and tea are examples of caffeinated beverages that should be drunk in moderation since they can increase the formation of stomach acid.

Cocoa:

There are substances in chocolate that could cause the lower esophageal sphincter to relax and cause acid reflux.

Spirits:

Alcohol can irritate the stomach lining, so limit or stay away from it.

CHAPTER THREE

fatty and fried foods:

Fried and high-fat foods might cause the stomach to empty more slowly and produce more acid.

Carbonated Drinks:

Carbonated beverages may be a factor in bloating and gas.

Consumption Patterns:

Little, Regular Meals:

Large, substantial meals may not be as taxing on the stomach as smaller, more frequent meals spread out throughout the day.

Chew Carefully:

Chew meals well to facilitate digestion and lessen the strain on the stomach.

Prevent Eating Late at Night:

If you want to reduce acid reflux, avoid eating right before bed.

Maintain Hydration:

Throughout the day, sip on lots of water to stay hydrated and promote good digestive health.

Individual Differences:

It's critical for people to be aware of how their bodies react and to pinpoint particular trigger foods that may exacerbate symptoms.

Maintaining a food journal might be useful for monitoring dietary trends and finding links between particular meals and worsening symptoms.

A licensed dietician or healthcare professional consultation can offer tailored advice based on dietary choices and specific medical problems.

Effective care of stomach ulcers is aided by dietary changes, medication, and lifestyle adjustments. Together with medical specialists, individuals should develop a customized, well-balanced eating plan that promotes healing and reduces the likelihood of symptom recurrence.

Modifications to Lifestyle

Apart from dietary modifications, lifestyle changes are essential for the management of stomach ulcers as they aid in the healing process, lessen inflammation, and stop the symptoms from recurring. For those who have stomach ulcers, the following lifestyle adjustments are crucial:

1. Quitting Smoking:

Smoking raises the possibility of complications and can slow the healing of ulcers. Giving up smoking improves general health and aids in ulcer healing.

2. Reducing Alcohol Consumption:

The stomach lining may get irritated by excessive alcohol drinking. Reducing alcohol consumption or abstaining from it lowers the chance of symptom aggravation.

3. Handling Stress:

Although it is not the direct cause of ulcers, stress can make symptoms worse. Use stress-reduction strategies like:

- Practices for deep breathing
- Meditating
- Yoga
- Frequent physical activity

4. Frequent Workout:

Regular physical activity improves digestion, lowers stress levels, and helps people maintain a healthy weight, among other health benefits.

5. Sufficient Sleep:

Make getting enough good sleep a priority because getting too little sleep can make you stressed out and negatively impact your general health.

6. Drinking plenty of water

Drink enough water to stay properly hydrated throughout the day. Maintaining the mucous lining of the stomach and promoting digestive health are two benefits of adequate water.

7. Adherence to Medication:

To reduce stomach acid and encourage the healing of ulcers, use prescription drugs—such as H2 blockers or proton pump inhibitors (PPIs) as instructed by medical professionals on a regular basis.

8. Steer clear of NSAIDs:

Avoid or use nonsteroidal anti-inflammatory medicines (NSAIDs) sparingly if at all feasible, as they may exacerbate the development of ulcers.

9. Controlling Weight:

Keep your weight in check with a well-balanced diet and frequent exercise. Being overweight might exacerbate acid reflux by putting more strain on the stomach.

10. Frequent Check-ins:

Keep up with routine follow-up visits with your doctors to discuss any new concerns, assess the healing of your ulcers, and modify your medication as needed.

11. Steer clear of triggers:

Recognize and stay clear of personal stressors that could exacerbate symptoms. This could involve particular meals, drinks, or pastimes.

12. Interaction with Medical Professionals:

Openly discuss any changes in symptoms, worries, or difficulties following the treatment plan with your healthcare providers.

13. Resources for Education:

To improve knowledge about managing stomach ulcers and making lifestyle changes, look for instructional materials or counseling.

14. Systems of Support:

Establish a network of friends and relatives to help you emotionally while you heal.

15. Consciously Consuming Food:

Eat mindfully by chewing your food slowly and appreciating every taste. This can facilitate digestion and lessen the stomach's workload.

16. Taking Caffeine Less Often:

Limiting caffeine intake may be helpful for some people, even if it's not always required to do so in order to ease stomach discomfort.

Patients with stomach ulcers should collaborate closely with medical professionals to customize lifestyle modifications to meet their unique requirements. Successful care of stomach ulcers is largely dependent on proactive engagement in lifestyle modifications, commitment to treatment programs, and regular communication.

Emotional Health and Coping Mechanisms

Managing the emotional side of things as well as the physical side of things is part of managing stomach ulcers. The following coping mechanisms and factors should be taken into account when treating stomach ulcers to preserve emotional well-being:

1. Learn for Yourself:

People can feel less anxious and more empowered to actively participate in their care if they have a thorough understanding of the nature of stomach ulcers, their causes, and the treatment approach.

2. Establish a Support Network:

Build a network of relatives and friends who can offer emotional support by sharing your experiences with them. Stress can be reduced by talking about worries and emotions.

3. Seek Expert Assistance:

If you're having trouble managing with emotions, think about seeing a mental health expert, like a therapist or counselor.

4. Mind-Body Methodologies:

To reduce stress and enhance mental health, try mind-body practices like mindfulness, deep breathing, or meditation.

5. Communicate Your Feelings:

Give yourself permission to feel everything, including fear, grief, and frustration. Restraining one's emotions might lead to further stress.

6. Establish sensible objectives:

Establish attainable objectives for yourself in terms of everyday living and controlling the physical components of the illness. Honor modest accomplishments and advancements.

7. Remain Upbeat:

Maintain an optimistic outlook. Try to find delight in everyday tasks and concentrate on the things you can manage.

8. Take It Slowly:

Don't take on more than you can handle. To lessen stress, divide larger jobs into smaller, more manageable steps.

9. Reduce the Overload of Information:

While being educated is crucial, try to avoid being overly exposed to material that could worry you unnecessarily.

10. Participate in Support Groups:

Joining an online or local support group can help those going through similar struggles by allowing them to share their stories and provide encouragement.

11. Adjust to Shifts in Lifestyle:

Recognize and constructively adjust to required lifestyle adjustments. Adopt a healthy diet and partake in activities that enhance your general state of wellbeing.

12. Take Care of Yourself:

Make self-care activities that relax and make you happy a priority. This could be engaging in hobbies, reading, going on nature walks, or watching a beloved film.

13. Maintain Contact:

Keep in touch with your loved ones, even if it's only virtually. Emotional health depends on social support.

14. Track Negative Ideas:

Keep an eye out for negative ideas and counter them with uplifting statements. Engage in self-compassion.

15. Honor Advancement:

Celebrate your successes and advancements in the treatment of your stomach ulcers. Acknowledge and value the efforts you are putting out.

CHAPTER FOUR

16. Think About Expert Advice:

Seeking the assistance of a mental health professional can help if stress or anxiety overwhelm you and can offer coping mechanisms and support.

17. Writing a Journal:

Write down your ideas and emotions in a diary. This can be a means of tracking your experience and providing an emotional outlet.

Managing stomach ulcers requires a comprehensive strategy that takes mental and physical health into account. It's critical to practice self-compassion, ask for help when you need it, and give priority to the pursuits that lead to a happy, healthy living.

Adopting lifestyle behaviors and habits that support a healthy digestive tract and reduce risk factors for ulcer formation are key to preventing stomach ulcers. The following are important precautions:

1. H. Prevention of H. pylori Infection:

Hygiene Practices: To lower the risk of Helicobacter pylori (H. pylori) infection, wash your hands thoroughly and practice excellent hygiene.

2. Usage of Medication:

Use of NSAIDs: Aspirin, ibuprofen, and naproxen are examples of nonsteroidal anti-inflammatory medicines (NSAIDs) that should be avoided whenever possible since they raise the risk of stomach ulcers.

3. Nutritional Habits:

Balanced Diet: To promote general digestive health, adopt a diet high in fruits, vegetables, whole grains, and lean proteins.

4. Reducing Foods That Irritate:

Eat Less or Stay Away from Spicy and Acidic Foods: Foods that are acidic, spicy, or irritate the stomach lining should be avoided.

5. Tobacco and Alcohol:

Moderate Alcohol Intake: Restrict alcohol intake to a minimum because too much of it can irritate the lining of the stomach.

Quit smoking: Smoking increases the risk of complications and can delay the healing of ulcers.

6. Handling Stress:

Stress Reduction Techniques: To lessen emotional stress, engage in stress-reduction practices like yoga, deep breathing exercises, meditation, or mindfulness.

7. Frequent Workout:

Physical Activity: To enhance digestive health and general well-being, get frequent exercise.

8. Drinking plenty of water

Sufficient Water Intake: Throughout the day, make sure you drink enough water to stay hydrated. Keeping the stomach's mucous lining in tact is facilitated by adequate hydration.

9. Frequent Examinations:

Health Screenings: See your doctor on a regular basis to assess your general health and rule out any risk factors.

10. Controlling Weight:

Sustain a Healthy Weight: To sustain a healthy weight, lead a healthy lifestyle that incorporates frequent exercise and a balanced diet.

11. Prevent Excessive Medication Use:

Limit Your Medication Use: Take prescription and over-the-counter pain medicines exactly as prescribed; don't use them for longer than necessary.

12. Limit your intake of coffee.

Moderate Caffeine Consumption: Avoid consuming too much caffeine as this can increase the formation of stomach acid.

13. Resources for Education:

Remain educated: Keep yourself educated on the causes of stomach ulcers and take the suggested precautions.

14. Handling of Concomitant Disorders:

Handle Underlying diseases: Collaborate with healthcare professionals to properly manage any underlying diseases you may have, such as GERD or other digestive disorders.

15. Probiotics:

Probiotic Foods: To support gut health, think about incorporating foods high in probiotics into your diet, like yogurt with living cultures.

16. Moderately Hot Meals:

Moderation with Spices: If you're a fan of spicy cuisine, try to limit your intake and observe how your body reacts.

17. Early Intervention:

Quick Medical Attention: If you have symptoms that don't go away or think you could have a stomach ulcer, get help right away. Complications can be avoided with early action.

A combination of risk factor awareness, healthy lifestyle choices, and quick symptom care can help prevent stomach ulcers. For individualized advice and recommendations, those with particular concerns or risk factors should speak with healthcare professionals.

CONCLUSION

Finally, it should be noted that stomach ulcers are a prevalent but treatable digestive system illness. Nonsteroidal anti-inflammatory drug (NSAID) use and Helicobacter pylori infection are two of the many potential causes, however there are effective management and preventative techniques.

Stomach ulcer formation and recurrence can be avoided by following a healthy lifestyle, eating a balanced diet, minimizing stress, and avoiding triggers. Successful treatment and the avoidance of complications like bleeding or perforation depend heavily on early detection and timely medical intervention.

A comprehensive strategy for controlling stomach ulcers combines medication, dietary changes, lifestyle improvements, and mental well-being techniques. Overall well-being is influenced by proactive health practices, following treatment regimens, and scheduling routine check-ups with medical professionals.

Those who are having symptoms or who may develop stomach ulcers should consult a healthcare provider. A healthcare provider can offer tailored advice based on the individual's circumstances. People can effectively manage stomach ulcers and lead healthy, fulfilling lives with the right care and attention.

THE END